Nature's Miracle
Fever Reducer
Lemongrass

NATURE'S MIRACLE
FEVER REDUCER

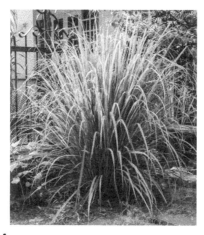

Lemongrass

GINGER GRASS/CITRONELLA
Jamaican Fever Grass

BOTANICAL NAME: *Cymbopogon Citratus*

EFELIN D. WILLIAMS

XULON PRESS

Xulon Press
2301 Lucien Way #415
Maitland, FL 32751
407.339.4217
www.xulonpress.com

Printed in the United States of America

Paperback ISBN-13: 978-1-6322-1254-2
Ebook ISBN-13: 978-1-6322-1255-9

TABLE OF CONTENTS

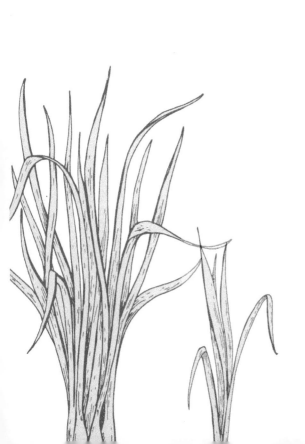

Disclaimer

Although I know, without a doubt, that Lemongrass has never hurt anyone, there are no side effects that I have ever experienced from using this herb whether from my backyard or from the teabags I purchased in the supermarkets, I have chosen to write a disclaimer. We are living in a country that encourages freedom of speech but you never know when someone may choose to twist the truth for their own benefit.

Upon reading this book, please do not "take my words" for it and start drinking Lemongrass. I must insist that you check with your Medical Doctor before drinking the Lemongrass tea as I am not a licensed physician. In the United States, only a Licensed Physician has the right, by law, to prescribe medication. I am certainly not recommending or prescribing Lemongrass tea, but merely stating the facts as I have experienced this miracle herb.

However, I must state that everything I have stated in my book is what I have experienced over these years and I do hope I will be able to help someone. Be safe.

Efelin Williams

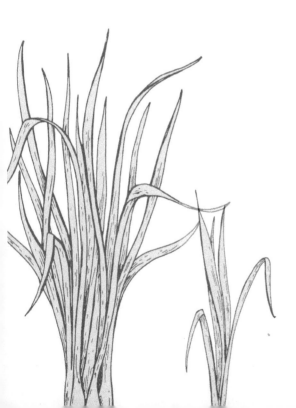

DEDICATION

I WOULD LIKE TO DEDICATE THIS BOOK TO these persons who have helped me to recognize the remarkable value of the Lemongrass plant. The amazing results I have had using this grass for not only myself, but also family members, friends and some of my patients as they experienced various illnesses has moved me to share my experience with others.

Firstly, Mrs. Mighty, who reminded me that I could use lemongrass to get my daughter's fever down when she came off the respirator after nine (9) days being intubated. She had a fever of 103 degrees although she was given various antibiotics during several days of hospitalization stay.

Secondly, the Mexican Plant Nursery owner, Luis, whom I met by chance one afternoon after a long day's work when I chose to drive through an unfamiliar neighborhood. My tour led me to pass by a nursery in Okeechobee. As I saw the plants and flowers, I felt a magnet as I passed by, which compelled me to make a U-turn and stop by to purchase plants and flowers.

Thirdly, Mrs. Miller, who gave me the esteemed opportunity to share with her my experiences of using lemongrass on more than one occasion to get better from different ailments. By sharing with her she was able to guide her son, who went to the Emergency Room when he felt he had contracted COVID-19. The 40-year-old young man was tested on Wednesday, April 22, 2020, prescribed antibiotics and sent home. It is now five days and he has not received the result of his COVID-19 test. However, his condition has greatly improved since he started drinking Lemongrass tea twice per day.

I pray this book will help others with similar illnesses to get well and indeed, save some lives.

Effelin D. Williams

INTRODUCTION

AS I WATCH THE NEWS INTENTLY DAY after day, I have a difficult time fighting back the tears when I hear that so many people are dying. Scientists and Medical staff throughout the United States are trying desperately to find a cure for this virus that is killing people across nations. In one particular case when I heard that there was someone still trying to get his temperature down after being discharged from the hospital, I relived the painful ordeal I went through when my own daughter was on a respirator for nine (9) days. She was being prepared to be discharged from the hospital with a temperature of 103 degrees when my friend suggested that she drink some lemongrass tea.

It is no wonder I sit here today, trying to express my sincere sympathy to the millions of families who are mourning the loss of their loved ones. I have had close relatives and friends who lost their children, and on each occasion, the pain I felt was beyond imagination, knowing that another mother is experiencing the horror of burying her child. The horror of burying a child does not seem to be the "perfect" order of how life should be; but it happens all the time, parents often bury their children, and it hurts!

While I continue to pray earnestly for the end of this pandemic, I wish to assist in whatever way I can, since I am now unable to be in the first line of duty because of my own illness. I wish you God's Grace and Mercy as we patiently wait on his pardon and to heal his land.

Chapter 1
GROWING UP WITH
NATURAL HERBS

AS A YOUNG CHILD I GREW UP AROUND adults who were very knowledgeable on the various herbs to use for the different ailments that we had. The family doctor saw me only when my tonsils were inflamed. Even then, I knew that I could gargle with warm salted water, and how soothing that treatment was! The older I became, the more I appreciated herbal treatment, because I have never had an allergic reaction to any of the herbal treatments that I was given by my parents.

A very common herb used by my mother was the Fevergrass or Lemongrass as I learned it is called quite late in my life. I was on my way home one Friday afternoon after a very interesting work-week. Usually, I turned left to go on the highway, but for some unknown reason, when I got to the stop sign, something possessed me to turn right. So I did. I checked my car to ascertain that there was enough gas in the event I made a turn that took me to the middle of nowhere. I kept questioning myself as I drove along the countryside, wondering why I chose to take a route I knew nothing about at that late time of day when it would soon get dark. However, it was refreshing to view the plants and flowers along the wayside, and I picked up some ideas for my own garden as I drove along. I also looked out for unusual animals, hoping desperately that I would see a deer.

I finally ended up in Okeechobee, and I suddenly saw a Plant Nursery as I drove by. Curiosity, as well as my love for plants and flowers, got the better of me, so I made a U-turn and drove into the parking lot. A very nice man came out and walked me through the nursery showing off the various plants and flowers he had, some of them I had not seen before. Suddenly, l saw a large pot with Fevergrass and I exclaimed: "Fevergrass". The owner, Luis, said to me in a kind tone of voice: "The botanical name is *Cymbopogon Citratus*", quite a mouthful for me, as I have always had a lisp, from sucking my tongue as a little girl.

"Oh, I exclaimed, thanks for telling me that, I had no idea what the correct name was". I have always been a sponge for knowledge and I really appreciated the botanical name of such a valuable plant because I love it and know how beneficial it is to my health. Luis then said, excitedly:

"Let me tell you a little story. About a year ago, a man came by and said he had Leukemia and the doctor gave him six months to live. I told him about the usefulness of the Lemongrass and he bought a plant. About four months after he came back to thank me. He said that he drank a cup of Lemongrass tea every night and when he went back to his doctor for his check-up there was no cancer. The doctor was surprised. He asked him what he did and he told him about the Lemongrass tea".

"Really now", I said to Luis, who was bursting with excitement as he boasted about the wonders of the Lemongrass plant. Of course I knew about Lemongrass and used it prior, but I had no idea it could cure cancer.

Luis' story caused me to reflect on how my parents used Lemongrass every time any of their children got a fever. I also recalled when my daughter was sick in the hospital and Mrs. Mighty asked: "Why don't you give her some Lemongrass tea, Efelin? You see, my daughter was on a respirator for nine (9) days. Even after she was taken off the respirator, she had a fever of 103 degrees and she was about to be discharged with the fever. I told Mrs. Might that I would not know where to get any Fevergrass and she said: "I have some at home". I begged her to make some tea and bring it into the hospital for her; while I stayed by her bedside and kept an eye on her.

When my friend returned with the Lemongrass tea, my daughter was given one cup. Mrs. Mighty prepared the tea with ginger in it and poured it in a thermos. After my daughter drank the tea, her temperature was normal when the nurse returned to check her vitals prior to being discharged. Thank God for his saving grace. Thank God for my friend. I will always hold her dear to my heart.

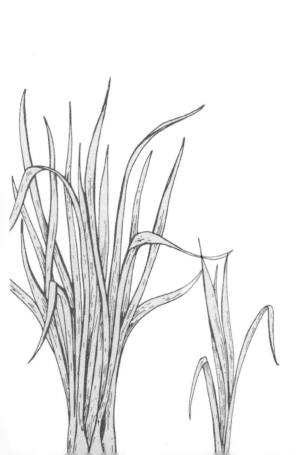

Chapter 2
ABNORMAL MAMMOGRAM

IN 2008 I DID MY ANNUAL MAMMOGRAM and the radiologist found a lump which was suspicious. My gynecologist told me to do an Ultrasound of my breast so that they could rule out cancer. Confused, frightened and determined not to be a victim of cancer, I decided right then and there that I was going to fight. My mother did not have any cancer, I said, so I know I do not, and will not have cancer.

Remembering what I learned from Luis, on my way home, I stopped at the health food store and picked up a box of Lemongrass tea bags. Yes, by then I had researched Lemongrass, this wonder healing plant, and discovered that it was sold in tea bag form so it was very convenient to keep in the kitchen. I recalled, quite vividly, what Luis told me about the man who was diagnosed with Leukemia. That very night when I learned of my diagnosis, I started to drink Lemongrass tea every night, just like the patient with Leukemia did.

When I returned to my doctor for the result of the Ultrasound, the lump was seen so I was scheduled for a biopsy. By then, I was not afraid. Not even for a single second did I think that I had cancer in my breast, because I knew for sure that the Lemongrass would work. I must confess though, that even without the Lemongrass, I have a very deep faith in God that he protects me from all ills. I have proved him so many times, whenever I go to God in prayer; he has always come through for me, undoubtedly. If I do not get what I ask him for, I know for sure he does not want me to have what I want, but what he desires for my life. So I placed my entire health in his hands and waited patiently on him. I was never stressed or afraid.

Chapter 3

BIOPSY APPOINTMENT

Upon my arrival at the surgery center for the biopsy, I joyfully went inside, although I was scheduled for a "hearing" at work immediately following the biopsy. Yes, when it rains, it pours, always in my life, but the fact that I am able to share this with you now, shows that God has always carried me through the storms, no matter how rough they are.

The nurse at the surgical center checked me in and I was sent to the room where the doctor would perform the biopsy. While I was lying on the table, the doctor and nurse kept looking at the previous ultrasound, then back at the screen on which my breast appeared. The doctor was looking at the Ultrasound that was taken previously of my left breast, while examining my left breast and looking on the monitor, trying to locate the lump. The nurse asked me my name and age to ascertain that I was the right patient. I verified my name and date of birth and she looked puzzled.

"There is no lump", the doctor said. I smiled and replied:

"Well, I have been praying", quite matter-of-factly, as if to say, what did I expect but answered prayers? And believe me, that was exactly what I expected.

The nurse responded:

"Well if you have been praying, it is not there. So many patients lie on that bed and say they have been praying, and there was no lump. I have seen this all the time".

For me, that was just another confirmation that miracles are still happening. Yes, God is still in the miracle business. You see, he loves us all. Remember, we are created in His own image, and as long as we follow his will for our lives, then we will definitely be blessed.

Chapter 4
GROWING LEMONGRASS
IN MY BACKYARD

SINCE THEN I HAVE ALWAYS PLANTED
Lemongrass in my backyard. I had three pots of Lemongrass,
and one day, I became frantic when someone who assisted
me with trimming the plants got rid of one pot of my pre-
cious Lemongrass. I hurried to Home Depot to replace the
lemongrass but they were out of stock. I finally asked my
neighbor for a plant and we shared experiences of how the
plant has helped our families and friends.

My daughter has also been planting this wonder tea
bush in her yard. However, during the winter months
she has to take the plant inside her house since the plant
does not do well in cold weather. You see, if you have children in the house they often get fevers, and Lemongrass
is a quick fix. It also provides a fresh aroma in the house[1]
while it cleanses the air which is
why I have now placed a pot of
Lemongrass in my house to keep
the air fresh.

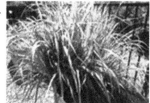

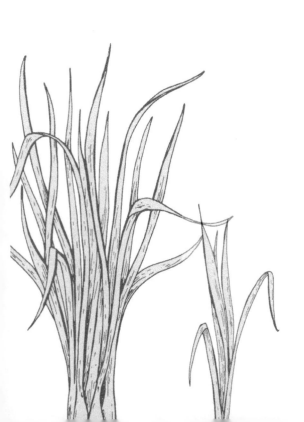

Chapter 5

PROPERTIES OF LEMONGRASS

So what is Lemongrass? Lemongrass is a plant that has antifungal and antibacterial properties.[2] My research on this wonder plant led me to discover the various properties of Lemongrass. Keeping a plant in your garden or in a pot in the house allows you to have the best medicine possible at your finger-tips. In the event you get a fever, there is no need to run to the pharmacy to purchase over-the-counter drugs that usually have side effects; some of which are deadly. So a cup of lemongrass tea can keep the temperature down until you are able to get to your physician.

RELIEVES PAIN & SWELLING

Just now I am reading that this supergrass relieves pain.[3] If Lemongrass can relieve pain and swelling, why should I take Opioids for pain when Lemongrass is a remedy that I do not even have to ingest? Just rubbing Lemongrass on the area where you are feeling pain will soothe the pain. It can also be used for swelling. Since the outbreak of

COVID-19, I started drinking Lemongrass tea at least once a day in order to boost my immune system.

I suffer from Chronic Regional Pain Syndrome and I gave credit to the warm weather for the improvement in the pain level I now feel. However, comparing last summer to this spring I realized that I had a lot more pain even in the summer last year than I have this spring–I know now that the only difference between the two seasons is I did not drink Lemongrass last summer, but because of the outbreak of COVID-19, I decided to boost my immune system with the Lemongrass. So yes, it certainly helps with pain. As for the swelling in my left ankle, it is gone down although my left foot and toes still hurt. Hip, hip, hooray!

On September 21, 2020 I fell in my backyard. Yes, although I suffer from Chronic Regional Pain Syndrome (CRPS), I do push myself to go out in the backyard to look for my land turtle that I named Sadie, and the squirrels and the rabbits as they search for food. Occasionally, I would see a butterfly or two, nesting on my blooms. I refuse to give up the pleasure of seeing the birds; lovingly feeding their young ones so I cheat on myself sometimes, not realizing that one day I would pay the price, and a high price it was.

As I walked from the sliding door to go into the garden, my foot compensated on the other leg to balance myself and my right knee made a cracking sound. "This is the end of me now". I thought to myself as I fell on my right hip. I was in total shock to see how easy it is to go from one happy moment to experiencing absolute fear in the blink of an eye. Unbelievable!

Too shock to do anything; I sat on the ground for a while, wondering what I should do. If I called 911, I told myself that would, of course, create too much excitement. So I sat there, not wanting to know too soon whether my right knee was worse than the left ankle. As soon as my left ankle twisted, I felt a sharp pain from my little toe shooting up to my groin. Frightening thoughts flooded my mind. Will I be going through the pain and suffering I have been experiencing for a longer time? Is anything broken? Will I be able to walk when I get up? How will I manage on my own if I cannot walk?

Shattered with fear, and overwhelmed with anxiety, I reached for the cell phone in my pocket and took a picture of myself on the ground. I just had to tell someone that I fell and I really wanted someone to pray for me that I was not going to be laid-up at this time in my life when I am just trying to embrace the joy of reduced pain. I sent the picture to my niece, who is a deacon, and asked her to say a prayer for me. She called and assured me that she would definitely pray for me. Then I was alerted by the neighbor who was plunging their sewage. And yes, my adrenalin took over. So I pushed up myself on my arms, carefully trying to test my legs before getting up, making sure that I did not hurt myself further in the process. I probably would not have moved just yet but I was definitely forced to once the smell of the sewage caught my nostrils.

Thankful that I could walk, I carefully went into my house and took two icepacks form the refrigerator and placed one on my knee and the other on my ankle. There was no swelling, just pain. Surprisingly, although I was in pain, it was more like an eight, instead of a ten as I experienced on previous occasions when I fell. I was not sure whether to be happy or sad; the fact that I was not feeling excruciating pain was of some concern, knowing that I have CRPS and other neurological problems. Anyways, I was extremely thankful that I could not only get up from the ground without help, but I could actually walk. Praise God!

I sat for a while putting ice on my knee and my ankle every 15 minutes. I then decided to call the nurse at my Insurance Company to get some advice on the best step to take. I was certainly afraid of going to the Emergency Room, considering that COVID-19 is so prevalent. The very kind nurse patiently listened to me then told me that the best advice she can give was that I should go to the Emergency Room to be checked out, especially since I heard the cracking sound in my right knee. I reminded her about the pandemic and she maintained that going to the Emergency Room would be the right thing to do. "How about the Walk-In Clinic?" I inquired. "There is one very close to me". Again, the nurse told me that it would be best for me to go to the Emergency Room. I told her "yes, I will go". Yeah, right! By the time I hung up I had already decided that it would be foolhardy to walk into an emergency room and get COVID-19 if I didn't have to go. So I stayed home, continued to use ice, fifteen minutes on and fifteen minutes off.

Before going to bed I took out my cane and my walker in preparation for the worse. I was not sure what to expect after inflammation sets in. I went to sleep early since I couldn't do much and I was afraid of hanging my feet down and causing them to get swollen. At approximately 10:00 p. m., I awoke to go to the bathroom. Ooops! My knee was as big as a basketball, but there was very mild pain. Unbelievable! This was not the first time I was having a sprained joint, yet this is the first time that I was not in excruciating pain. I marveled at the possible reasons and then the thought came to me like a light bulb. Ever since COVID-19 started back in February I have been taking lemongrass to prevent myself from getting the virus. Then I recalled that one of the benefits of lemongrass is it relieves pain and swelling. So, my ankle was twisted, but not swollen. My knee was swollen but there was no pain.

I sat on the side of my bed for a while, examining my body and couldn't understand why this time around my symptoms were so different. Yet, I was elated that I was not in excruciating pain and I could help myself around the house. In all my years of getting injuries, this was my first experience with pain lower than ten. I was able to get to the bathroom without incident and was overjoyed at the fact that I could get the ice from the refrigerator and ice my knee before going back to sleep.

Since my knee was very swollen, I texted my friend who lives five minutes from my house, asking her to take me to the emergency room the next day. I assured her though that because of the pandemic, if the swelling went down I would not be going. I then heated up a cup of lemongrass tea and drank it before returning to bed, hoping that all the swelling would disappear before I woke up. Unfortunately, there was still swelling on Tuesday, September 22, but not as big as it was during the night.

Finally, I went to the emergency room. My friend wanted to stay but she was not allowed because of COVID-19 so she left me there and told me to call her and update her on what was happening. When the X-ray was done I had a sprained ankle, a sprained groin and a sprain knee. My pain-level was, and is still surprisingly below what I usually feel under similar circumstances and I attribute this to the fact that I have been drinking lemongrass daily since February.

LEMONGRASS PLANT AS A MOSQUITO REPELLANT

I live opposite an area that gathers water in the blocked trench on the median whenever it rains. So whenever the water sits there for a while, there is an infestation of mosquitoes in the area. I have no screen on my front door so as soon as I open it the mosquitoes fly in and nothing is more annoying!

On one occasion I was trying to watch TV when I heard one of my unwelcomed guests buzzing at my ear. Since I had nothing in my house to kill mosquitoes I thought of using some dried lemongrass leaves to burn them out. I was very cautious though, since I had never tried this before. I placed some of the dried lemongrass leaves from the plant I have growing in my backyard in a cookie can and lit it, allowing the smoke to fill the air. That was done approximately one month ago and up to the time of writing this page I have not seen any mosquitoes.

Since then, I have done some research and found that Lemongrass Essential Oil can be used as a repellant. The oil is very acidic and in one study in which several species of mosquitoes was used, 95% of the mosquitoes were repelled.[4] So, not only is the lemongrass plant good for medicinal purposes, but it can also be used as a repellant. I will be treating myself to some essential oils for future use if I ever have mosquitoes in my house, but the dried leaves worked just fine when I had an emergency.

Knowing that the strong odor of lemongrass will get rid of the mosquitoes, I allow the steam to fill the air when I am making a pot of tea. The aroma is great, and there are no more mosquitoes around.

Helps with Anxiety

I am very concerned about the lives of people dying all over the world, and–I am especially concerned for my own family and friends. Usually I become very worried and over-whelmed with fear and anxiety. However, I am not anxious. I noticed that I even sleep more than usual. Up to a month ago I would be awakened at least twice every night to use the bathroom and sometimes I had to struggle to go back to sleep. Recently, I have been sleeping like a baby. The only thing I do differently is to drink at least one cup of Lemongrass tea every day. I often substitute the tea for water, not only because I like the taste, but also because I know that the virus is so deadly and I want to protect myself.

BUILDING MY IMMUNE SYSTEM DURING COVID-19

Knowing as much as I do about the various ways in which I can use Lemongrass, I regularly drink the tea. After drinking a cup of tea in the morning, I add more water and lemon to make enough and continue drinking it throughout the day. On occasions I add Tumeric to ward off inflammation, just in case I come in contact with the virus. There is a better chance to fight the virus if you have a strong immune system, regardless of your age.

INGREDIENTS FOR LEMONGRASS TEA

The ingredients for Lemongrass Tea is below:

3 stalks Lemongrass

2 cups water

1 lemon

2 Tablespoons ginger powder or grated ginger

1 Tablespoon turmeric (optional)

METHOD

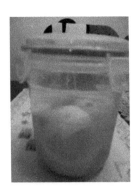

Wash lemongrass stalks and chop them up in small pieces. Slice one lemon. Add the chopped stalks to water and bring it to a boil. Allow it to seep while adding ginger, tumeric and sliced lemon pieces. This should be served warm, since the virus does not thrive in heat. You may add honey if you are allowed to use honey, but sugar should be avoided.

How this mixture can help during COVID Virus

Usually, if you go to the Emergency Room when you recognize the symptoms, the test is done and you wait a few days to get the result. During the waiting period your symptoms can be greatly improved if you drink this mixture. So, spread the word, and prevent the symptoms from getting critical. Save a life!

Andrae's Recovery

Earlier I mentioned that Andrae was tested in the ER for COVID-19. Andrae quarantined himself for 14 days. During that time he drank a cup of Lemongrass tea in the mornings and another cup at nights. I was blessed with a phone call from his mom on Wednesday, May 13, 2020 thanking me for my suggestion that he should drink the Lemongrass tea. Andrae followed up with a phone call thanking me and raving about his recovery, and I encouraged him to write about his journey through the contraction and the healing process of COVID-19 so that others may benefit from the steps he took to heal himself. He will be returning to work with a new attitude as he practices social distancing, wearing his mask and hand sanitization. Hopefully he will donate his plasma so that he can save the lives of others.

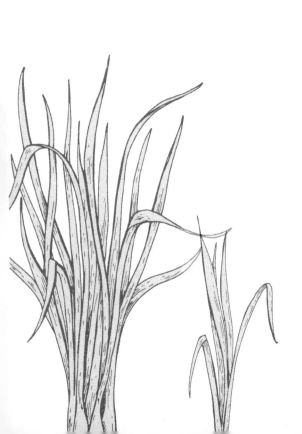

Chapter 6
AVAILABILITY OF LEMONGRASS

LEMONGRASS PLANT IS AVAILABLE AT Amazon, Etsy, Lowes, Home Depot and Walmart, to name a few places. It is also available in tea bag form at the West Indian stores and Bravo. There is also a Lemongrass Outlet where you can get amazing discounts. So protect yourself from viruses, keep your temperature down if you get a fever, and share your knowledge with someone else whose life you may save.

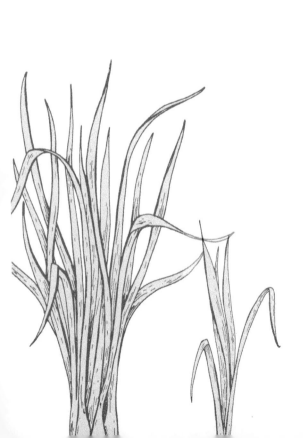

Acknowledgements

I WOULD LIKE TO ACKNOWLEDGE ALL MY friends and relatives who encouraged me along this journey. A special thank you to my cousin, Shevannese Mighty for being my second pair of eyes. Your attention to detail, your pleasant demeanor and your calm spirit is such a positive influence on my life.

To my life-long friend, Carmen Dennis, thanks for the push you gave me when I felt weary. I do hope you will be able to get the plant to grow in your house. The weather where you are in Canada is so cold, but when you visit me in Sunny South Florida I will ensure that you get a taste of my delicious Fevergrass tea just like back in the good old days.

I will be forever grateful to the staff of Salem Author Services for their patience with me as I continued adding to my manuscript when I discovered more ways to use the Lemongrass plant. I really appreciate you all.

My Special gratitude also to Brenda Dempsey, Michael Dempsey and Jeanette Dean for believing in me and trusting me completely to share my story with others, while you enjoy the benefits of using Lemongrass. I wish for you all continued health and wellness as you discover for yourselves how powerful this plant really is in maintaining your health and wellbeing.

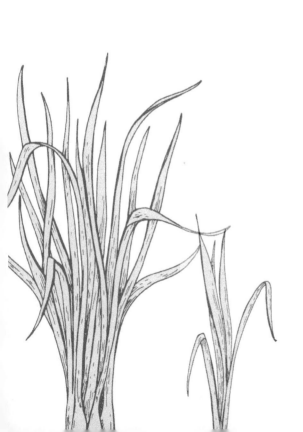

Bibliography

1   Keville, Kathi, *Aromatherapy: Lemongrass health, howstuffworks.com/wellness/natural-medicine/aroatherapy/aromatherapy.*

2   SimplyHealth. Today, 20 *-reasons–why-you-will-benefit-from-lemongrass.*

3   Yahoo Search Results Search.yahoo.com, *Healthline.com/health/fitness-exercise/essential-oils-for-sore-muscles#pain-and-swelling.*

4   https://mosquitoreviews.com/mosquito-repellents/lemongrass

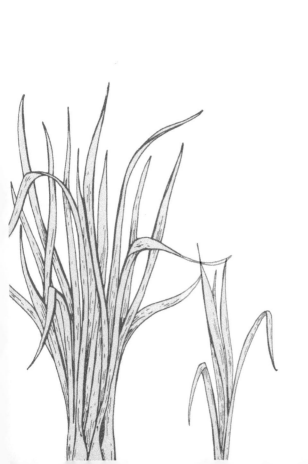

ABOUT THE AUTHOR

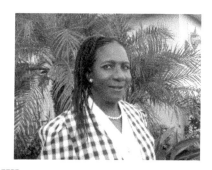

EFELIN WILLIAMS GRADUATED FROM THE University of the West Indies with a Business Studies Degree and a certificate in creative writing. She wrote several poems and her instructor was impressed by her imagination. She also completed a writing course at Nova Southeastern University. She has always had an interest in writing but was not sure how she could make a livelihood being a writer so she focused on gaining a Bachelors of Public Administration degree from Barry University and a Health Information Management degree from Broward College, where she served as Historian in Phi Theta Kappa. She worked for several years as a Medical Records Coordinator and also did Court Reporting. Now that she is retired she has the time to focus on her first love, writing, and with a desire to help people from all walks of life, wish to share her experiences with others in order to improve lives.

CPSIA information can be obtained
at www.ICGtesting.com
Printed in the USA
BVHW092022070522
636264BV00002B/7

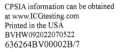